THE TEXT-BOOK OF WEIGHT-LIFTING

(ORIGINAL VERSION, RESTORED)

By

ARTHUR SAXON

Originally Published in 1910

PUBLISHED BY O'Faolain Patriot LLC, Copyright 2011
info@PhysicalCultureBooks.com
Published in the United States of America

ISBN-13: 978-1466466258

ISBN-10: 1466466251

To Order More Copies Visit: Physical Culture Books.com

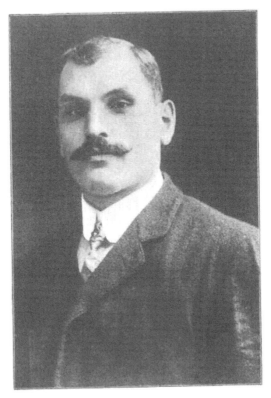

ARTHUR SAXON.

Finally, the publisher disclaims any and all liabilities arising from the use of any equipment featured in this book and makes no representations as to the utility, safety, or adequacy of the equipment generally or with respect to any specific purpose.

TABLEOFCONTENTS

CHAPTER I
Why Weight-lifting should be regarded as the first of all Sports and also as the best form of Physical Exercise

To my mind, every man should devote at least some small attention to Weight-lifting. I don't think that I have come to this conclusion simply because I myself have gained some distinction as a weight-lifter, but rather for the reasons set forth below.

First of all, why does a man learn to box? Well, because it is asserted that every man should learn how to defend himself in case of necessity. A good and sufficient reason, you will say.

The same may also be put forward as an excuse for learning wrestling and ju-jutsu no doubt, but I am inclined to fancy that the noble art would possibly be more useful than either.

As to fencing, club-swinging, etc., I know no reason for their practice except it be that of pleasure or a desire for physical exercise, which said reasons may be equally advanced for Weight-lifting, which it will, I think, be further readily admitted is the most sure and certain means of developing strength —a quality which would be most undeniably useful in any means of self-defence.

Now, beside all this, every man in every walk of life is certain, sooner or later, to be confronted with a heavy object, bulky or otherwise, which he strongly desires to lift.

This may occur both in his business and in his private life, and I am willing to bet that each and every man on such an occasion entertains a certain amount of regret for the wasted hours which he might have advantageously devoted to practise with weights.

Now, the chief objection which the opponents of Weight-lifting always advance is that it makes a man slow and cumbrous.

Further than that, it is and has been contended that by developing one's strength to the degree of coping with weights of two or three hundredweight, a man will transform himself into a species of clumsy elephant; a kind of navvy, who is able certainly to heave and push, but unable to do anything but that. In short, totally incapable of anything resembling delicacy or skill, and that, worst of all, he will only have so spoilt himself at the cost of a strained, weakened heart and a twisted, possibly ruptured, frame.

Very serious and crushing objections these, and quite sufficient to put any man off Weight-lifting altogether—supposing them to contain even a tittle of truth. But do they?

As to the stale old charge of slowness, this has been argued and discussed until it must be pretty nearly threadbare, but I do not remember ever to have come across any specified instance which those who make the assertion have ever attempted to quote in support of their case. Rather strange this, isn't it?

Again, while it is quite possible to point to several weight-lifters who are slow in movement, conception, and execution, compared with such a man as Tommy Burns, for instance, it will invariably be found that these men are naturally and constitutionally slow and cumbrous, and that, if their whole record is examined, that they have become far quicker men since they took up Weight-lifting than ever they were before.

Look at Hackenschmidt, for instance, or, for that matter, Lurich, or almost all of the big Continental wrestlers. These were, one and all of them, weight-lifters before they dreamt of becoming wrestlers. Can it be suggested that they are slow and cumbrous men, and will it not be considered not altogether unreasonable to suppose that some of their present quickness was developed—by their Weight-lifting experiences?

On one point most opponents, and even some advocates, of Weight-lifting appear to be agreed, that it would be foolish for a boxer to think of indulging in Weight-lifting exercises.

Now, I am not disposed to fall in with this opinion so easily. I boxed a man seriously on one occasion myself, but I think, perhaps, that I had better reserve that incident for the present, as I can't quote it very well in support of my opinion, especially as there are many others which will serve me better.

Jack Johnson, the big negro, is regarded by many people, not only as being fully the equal, but even possibly the superior of the great Tommy Burns himself, and yet Johnson is no mean weight-lifter. He even occasionally performs a bridging feat, that is to say, makes a bridge supporting men on his chest and stomach— a weight-lifting feat pure and simple.

Tommy Burns himself, who strongly deprecates all Weight-lifting exercises in his excellent "Scientific Boxing and Self-Defence," yet indirectly admits a. certain virtue in dumb-bells at all events, by holding them in his hands when punching the bag and also when going through his stomach exercises. He admits as much in his most interesting chapter on Training.

Tom Sayers is said to have developed his hitting powers by heaving bricks, just as Tom Cribb acquired his by heaving sacks of coal, both of which could be far more satisfactorily substituted by ring and flat weights.

Now, as to the delicacy of touch and skill business—well, the comparison of the weight-lifter with an elephant surely defeats its own ends, since, while the elephant is great at pulling and pushing weights, he is no less adept at picking up pins.

Delicacy of touch and quickness of eyesight and movement—well, let us take Professor Inch as an instance. Here is a man who has passed most of his life as a weight-lifter, and yet if there is a better nursery cannon player at billiards or a better " snap" rifle shot about, I should like to see him.

Doesn't nursery cannon striking demand the finest delicacy of touch imaginable? Must not a man, upon whose ability to bring down seagulls from a small rowing-boat, in a rough sea, you can safely lay ten to one, be possessed of an unerring sharpness of vision and an instinctive harmonious union of muscle, brain, and nerve?

This is, I think, the greatest virtue in Weight-lifting. In no other branch of athletics which I have been able to observe (and I have, I think, studied them all) is it so absolutely necessary for the whole body to move together, to co-ordinate itself so perfectly.

The opponents of Weight-lifting see only the slow pushing aloft of a heavy bar, and totally fail to notice the lightning rapidity with which this is "pulled in" to the shoulder, or with which the lifter gets "under" it. There are many movements in Weight-lifting which are every bit as quickly executed as any of those of a champion boxer.

Finally, as to the deleterious effects which the practice of lifting heavy weights are supposed to have on the general health and internal organism — well, you will, perhaps, allow me to instance my own case.

For the last fourteen years I have been regularly lifting weights of every description, and have, moreover, put up to arm's length, with one hand only, within 16 lbs. of the utmost weight that anybody else has ever jerked with both hands. (In fact, only one man, Josef Steinbach to wit, has ever lifted as much with both hands as I have with one.)

So that, according to the opponents of Weight-lifting, I ought to be more or less in a state of physical collapse, with a strained heart and twisted intestines; in short, I should really be steadily sinking one foot into the grave.

That is the theory, but what are the facts?

Will these opponents of Weight-lifting allege that any man other than a weight-lifter could have come whole out of my recent accident?

Would they imagine themselves to be possessed of such stamina, and to be sound in wind and limb, as to be able to endure being crushed under a platform—motor-car and passengers—of a total weight of close on 3 tons, and after a few months' attention in the way of bandages, splints, open-air life, etc. be in pretty nearly as good condition as they were before the accident?

My brother Kurt, who was also involved in the smash, certainly got off better than I did, but he nevertheless had a foot crushed and a few other injuries. In spite of these, however, he was at work again lifting weights and performing feats of strength within a week or so.

How's that for the weight-lifter's constitution?

Weight-lifting as a Test of Strength.

People are always arguing about the relative amount of strength possessed by different men; but when all other arguments are exhausted, they are compelled to come back to a comparison of the heaviest weight which each of the claimants can lift, and to decide finally on that basis.

In every other branch of athletics by which relative "strength" can be tested, " skill " enters so extensively into the question of pre-eminence as practically to reduce strength to a secondary consideration.

Now, skill enters into Weight-lifting as well. In fact, it dominates the situation quite as fully therein as it does in boxing or wrestling; but then, in

Weight-lifting, and in Weight-lifting alone, is skill synonymous with strength.

A really strong man who is unable to lift really heavy weights can only be described as a man who possesses possibilities of strength, while a man who can exceed 250 lbs. with either one or two hands (or even 200 lbs., supposing him to be a 9 to 10-stone man) is the fortunate possessor of real strength, having been endowed with actual power itself, which he has further acquired the ability to use.

Every normally sound and healthy man, whose doctor can assure him that his heart is sound, and who has attained the age of from sixteen to nineteen (according to the proportionate development he has attained at those ages), not only can, but should, enter upon some course of Weight-lifting or of exercises with weights.

Supposing him to entertain a strong ambition to gain distinction as a boxer, runner, or swimmer, it would not, I think, be advisable for him to overdo the business, but in either of such events he should at least select a few exercises and practise them seriously.

His choice of exercises will naturally be governed by the muscular groups which will be of most assistance to him in the branch of athletics he proposes eventually to shine, and he will, or should, confine his practice mainly to those exercises which will specially develop those very groups.

But, supposing him to be in any doubt in the matter, and not quite certain whether other exercises (such as will strengthen allied groups) would not be also beneficial, then would I advise him to apply for further advice to some instructor such as Professor Inch, for example, who can give him thoroughly expert advice on any point which may be troubling him.

In any case, however, I would recommend that application be made only to a thoroughly qualified man, one, indeed, who holds a diploma from the Inch Institute, since I can safely assert that any man who has gone through the course necessary to attain that distinction must be fully competent in every respect. When applying for such advice, it would be wise to state particularly the objects in view and the difficulties which assail the applicant, as the expert applied to would naturally need such information for his guidance.

CHAPTER II
Clean Lifting

IN England far more importance is attached to what is known as "clean" lifting than is the case elsewhere.

On the Continent of Europe particularly it does not matter much how a man gets his weight to his shoulder provided he "puts it away" all right afterwards.

The Continental weight-lifter has, of course, to "shoulder" his bell by the exercise of his own unaided strength, but he may lift it shoulder high with both hands, or by levering it up his body, according to the lift in question. But, as I shall deal with all these points in my chapter on Continental Lifting, I need not dwell further on the point here.

Clean lifting, however, since it was the method adopted at the old Amateur Championships, obtained thereby the seal of official approval, and will, I presume, always be esteemed the finest and fairest test in a contest between British weight-lifters.

There is no reason why anyone should object to this, as the clean " pull in " to the shoulder is a pretty and a skilful feat, demanding both strength and judgment, but I am inclined to fancy that the old " Four Championship Lifts," by which all British competitions used to be decided (when there were any) is distinctly susceptible of improvement.

First of all, because the invariable selection of these same four lifts circumscribed the weight-lifter. He rarely, if ever, troubled to practise any other lift, and, consequently, fell behind his Continental rival.

For I am positive that if a man wishes to excel at the game he must become an all-round lifter.

Almost every lift demands the full exercise of all the muscles. That will, I think, be admitted, as will also the fact that nearly every lift puts an extra strain on some one particular group.

So that, if a man practises thoroughly all-round lifting, he will equally develop every portion of his body, and thus be enabled to do better at the four "championship" lifts themselves than he could possibly hope were he to practise those four lifts only.

Then, in making a match or arranging a competition, a list could be prepared of the following :

Right and left hand clean; two dumb-bells clean; two-handed bar-bell clean; to the shoulder anyhow, and then one hand clean (which would cover the bent press); two hands to the shoulder anyhow and then clean; dumb-bell swing; right; left; and two-handed snatch.

There is a list of ten distinct all-round lifts, from which the contestants (or the governing body) could select six, which would be ample. The result would, I am convinced, provide a far more interesting contest than the old championship tournaments used to be.

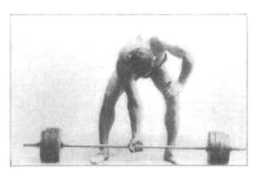

Position for One Hand Clean Pull In.

Ring weights, square weights, and dumb-bells held out at arm's length might, however, provide a welcome variation, and could be considered, as might also the bar-bell raised from the ground.

There are numerous other lifts, but I should be inclined to describe most of these as being more or less " trick " lifts, and, therefore, not such as could or should be introduced into a contest or tournament.

Nevertheless, I certainly think that at least six or seven lifts should be recognised as the only satisfactory minimum, and would strongly advise all my readers to make a point of steadily practising at least ten or twelve of the lifts I shall describe in this book.

By so doing, they will find that they will be able to add lbs. to their present records at even their own pet lifts, and that, in consequence, their physical strength and all-round vitality will be considerably improved.

The great thing, of course, is to attack and carry through each lift in the correct style, and though I may not hold world's records at every individual lift, I have, however, had sufficient experience of most of them to enable me to form a pretty accurate idea as to the best method of attempting them all, so that I do not think you will go very far wrong if you follow such advice as I am able to offer.

Single-handed Bar-bell Lift—clean all the way

Better results can always be obtained by using the bar-bell for the single-handed clean lift, since, owing to the length of the weight and the consequent more even distribution, the bell " springs " well from the ground, swings round better, and, therefore, can both be pulled in to the shoulder and started on its journey aloft without so much difficulty, lb. for lb.

In approaching this lift, the first thing to ascertain exactly is the centre of the bar, or (supposing a shot or sand-loaded bell be used, in which there may be some slight variation between the load in each sphere) the dead centre of the weight.

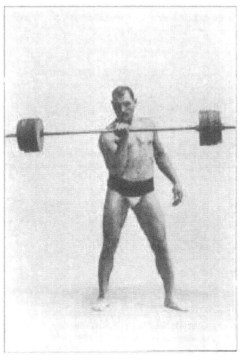

One Hand Clean Pull To
Turning to Shoulder

It is advisable, therefore, to mark the centre of the weight in such manner that it can be gripped at that point immediately, and without worry or fuss. For this reason alone (if there were no others), disc-loading bells should always be used, for with this kind the weights at each end must equalise, and the centre, therefore, can be always clearly marked beforehand.

Apart from this, no time is lost in adding or removing the discs, while, for some reason or other, there is far greater spring in a disc bell than in a shot or sand-loaded bell.

Having ascertained your centre, stand over the bar with your feet under it (so that it crosses your insteps), the feet being well apart and pointing outwards.

Stoop down, or rather sink down, as though you were just about to "sit" (but only go half-way), bending forward at the hips. Grip the exact centre of the bar firmly with your fingers underneath, and take a full deep breath, filling your lungs to the very limit. Your left hand (supposing this to be a right hand lift) should be pressed firmly against the bottom of your left thigh, just above the knee.

Then pull the bar straight up to your chin, at the same time pressing hard against your knee with your left hand, taking care that both movements are simultaneous. (See note below on " pulling in " at end of chapter.)

As soon as the bar has come right up to the chin, and it must come up straight and in one clean pull, stride out with the right foot, turning your hand over, so that the elbow comes directly under the bar, close to your side over your hip. This is another sharp movement, and it is as well to point out that no time should be wasted either in preparing to pull in or in turning the bell, as delay in either of these movements will assuredly spell failure.

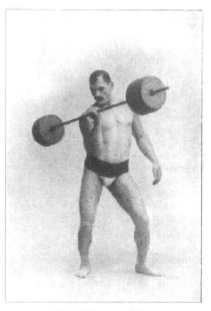

THE TWO-HAND "CLEAN" LIFT.
Elbow resting on hip, preparatory to bending ...... to get "under" the weight.

An Opinion on Contact

The Amateur Weight-lifting Championships must, I suppose, now be considered to be things of the past, so that there is, I believe, considerable doubt as to the actual limits of a perfectly clean lift. For instance, I have heard several authorities declare that a man who in pulling in, turning, or pressing his weight allows it to touch any part of his body save the hand lifting it, should be forthwith disqualified for that attempt.

This, I think, to be a very absurd stretching of the powers of a referee, for the slightest overswing of a bell might easily bring it into contact with the opposite shoulder without in any way yielding thereby assistance to the lifter.

A clean lift should, of course, not be steadied at any time by a touch from the other hand, but surely full discretion should be allowed to the judge in this matter! He could easily decide whether any further contact was accidental or willful, and also whether such contact was calculated to help the lifter unduly, and give his decision accordingly without being bound down by any too stringent ruling.

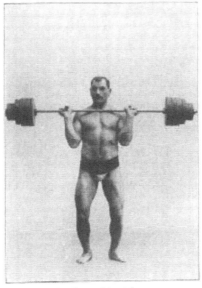

Continental Two-Hand Lift.
Pulled in and ready for jerking.

The Clean Press from the Shoulder

After the bar-bell has been " pulled in" and turned, there are two ways (according to English methods) by which it can be sent away to arm's length, viz., the " bent press " and the "jerk." As the first, however, was the one adopted in English Championship lifts, I propose to deal with that first, especially as a far heavier weight can be dealt with in that fashion. A heavier weight, indeed (as I shall show later on) than can be pulled clean in to the shoulder itself, single-handed.

For the bent or body press, with the hand turned and elbow in a direct line below, turn the bell steadily, working the elbow round until the latter rests on the hip itself, and gradually let your body fall away sideways and slightly forwards.

By the way, there is a point here at which my own methods run directly opposed to those generally in use. I believe my own to be the best way, but have heard so many people declare that I have only proved it to be so because of some peculiarity in my build, that I feel that I should mention other lifters' ways as well as my own.

They swing their bar round as they sink their bodies, commencing the latter operation with the bar at right angles to the shoulder. By so doing, they are performing three movements at the same time— sinking the trunk sideways and forward, turning the body, and turning the bell—a triple feat which I fancy tends to loss of all control over the weight.

Personally, I turn my weight first, so that it is almost parallel with my body, before I allow the latter to sink, and this, I believe, makes me master of the situation far more easily.

One other point, by the way, which I have overlooked is the absolute necessity of getting one's feet into the right position before sinking away from the weight. With the weight at the shoulder, you are better situated than at any other time to get your balance securely; any subsequent attempt to shift same can only invite failure.

There are, of course, no rules for this same placing of the feet. A weight-lifter will naturally do this to suit himself. The illustrations will give him a fairly clear idea of the pose, but the distance apart, etc., must be as he feels himself most comfortable.

When sinking forward, the disengaged hand or arm should be placed on the left knee, and is by some lifters slid across the knees, so that, while the elbow rests on, say, the left knee, the hand is pressed against the right thigh. I do not recommend this, nor do I advise placing the hand on the ground, as in both cases it must leave its first support, as the body subsequently straightens itself and cannot fail thereby to endanger the preservation of one's balance.

In pressing the arm straight from the bent position, always endeavour to keep your elbow supported on your hip bone as long as possible. Remember that your bones have been constructed to stand a greater strain than your muscles.

You can, indeed, by gradually sinking lower and raising your shoulder somewhat more than half-straighten your arm without allowing the latter to lose the support of your side, and, in any event, by a steady concentration of all your muscles, have so far straightened it as to have gained a good steady impetus towards the final straight push by arm strength only.

When the elbow finally leaves the side it should swing slowly round to the back until the shoulder is " locked," thus securing a position from which one's entire muscular strength can be utilised for the final effort. The " locking " proceeds slowly as the arm goes through the final straightening process. The most critical point of the whole lift is when the elbow leaves the-side, and unless all one's efforts are concentrated on the correct performance of the movement, control is apt to be lost.

When the arm is at last straight, you should be able to draw a. perfectly straight line from the centre of the bell, through your hand, down through both shoulders, and the left knee to the left foot.

If this position has been secured, dip the body slightly as shown, in order to come directly under the bar. You have only then to push off steadily from your left knee with your left hand, and you can stand erect with the lift accomplished.

As soon as you are sure of this, bring up your other hand, and so lower the bell first to your chest and then to the ground.

Final Hints

Many famous lifters will always advise you to keep the elbow well on the side (meaning thereby the apex of the hip bone). Personally, I prefer to take it further round, almost on to my back, as I find that by so doing I can not only lock my shoulder better before standing erect, but can also sink forwards rather than sideways.

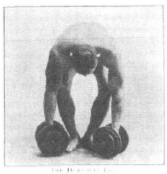

This last is, I think, an advantage, as I can get well under the weight better, and, moreover, do not cramp the muscles on my left side so much as I should were I to sink more to the left; so that, as I like to have the help of those muscles as well, I have no desire to cramp them more than I need.

Two final points. Supposing that during the course of your lift you find that you are losing control of your bell, endeavour first to regain it and proceed; but if this becomes difficult, drop the weight altogether and jump clear.

Then you will soon become aware that your strength is beginning to leave you from the moment you have pulled your weight in, and that it is advisable to get the lift over as soon as possible. Do not, however, on that account forget the proverb, "More haste, less speed "; but recollect rather that perfect balance must be preserved at all costs, and that any hurry in pressing which will disturb your control of the weight is a sheer waste of time and energy. Never take your eyes off the bell at any moment during the press.

One-handed Jerk from Shoulder

The other style of sending your bell to a straight arm and so standing erect is by " jerking " it.

In this lift, the legs come into play almost as much as the arm does, and the lift, to be successful, must be performed with the utmost rapidity.

With the bell " pulled in," bring your elbow slightly to the front. Look up and throw out your disengaged arm, so as to preserve your balance.

Split your legs slightly, say 15 to 18 inches, and then bend your knees a little and shoot up straight, so as to fling your arm up well off your hip. A slight second dip at the knees will enable you to straighten your arm, without much muscular effort in that limb, and you can rise erect with the arm in the same position as at the completion of the bent press.

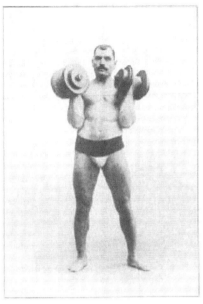

Two Bar-bell Lift.
(Pulled in English Style.)

Two-handed Bar-bell Lift

The bar-bell can be either pushed or jerked overhead with both hands, but as the former method is more common on the Continent than it is in this country, I propose dealing with it in my chapter on Continental Lifting.

To jerk the bell in the English method, the weight must first be pulled in clean to the shoulders, and in this case it is quite as important to mark the gripping places for each hand, as it is for the one hand in the single-handed lift.

These gripping places should be equidistant from the exact centre of the bar, and as far apart as

27

will bring your hands just outside your shoulders when the weight is pulled in.

Don't waste time playing with the bar in a stooping posture, but make up your mind that you are quite ready to lift; then go up to the bar, stand over it a moment, filling your lungs and stringing up your energies, stoop sharply down, grip it firmly and pull it up to your chin.

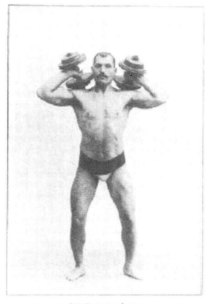

TWO IRON BELL LIFT
Pulled in resting on shoulders.
A good position at which to rest before overhead.

As it comes up, most weight-lifters take a slight forward and backward step with either foot, as they turn the bar in pulling in with a turn of the wrists and elbows, so as to bring these underneath the bell and at the same time sink the body a trifle, so as to

28

bring the abdomen under the weight as well. This movement and an extra final pull up, just as they are turning the weight, they claim to find of great assistance to them.

For my own part, however, I find this movement of the feet apt to disturb balance, besides (to my mind) distinctly ungainly. My brothers both step back with the right foot in pulling in, in spite of my protests. They have, indeed, to make two unnecessary movements, the backward step and the return one, in order to secure the "pause" position before jerking.

Once this is secured, as shown in photograph, take another deep breath, and again call on your muscles for the jerk aloft. Don't bend your back at any time during any part of the jerk itself, as this is almost certain to bring you down.

Now dip sharply beneath the bell, bending your knees outwards and straightening them even more sharply, throw your arms straight, quickly dipping again, so as to drop away from them as they go up. This will straighten them almost without calling heavily on the arm muscles. On no account jerk part of the way and push the rest. The arms must go straight from the throw-off, the shoulders merely aided solely by the second dip.

Then with arms erect, straighten legs and rise erect.

FOR EXHIBITION PURPOSES the bell may now be lowered to the back of the neck and again jerked aloft. The movement is practically the same, although a little more arm strength enters into the feat, which can be exerted more easily, owing to the more favourable position for that purpose.

Two Dumb-bells—Simultaneous Clean Lift

This, the last of the old championship four, is a much more difficult feat to some lifters than the two-handed bar-bell, although I believe that Mr. Caswell has lifted more in this lift (and with unequal dumb-bells to boot) than he could manage with the bar-bell.

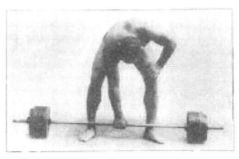

Different lifters use different methods of pulling in a pair of dumb-bells to the shoulders, and, honestly, since I have seen so many excellent performances with each method, I am somewhat loath to advise.

In any event, the best way to commence is to stand with heels together and bells close to the legs. Stoop down, bending at the hips and knees, and grasp the bells firmly close to the front discs or spheres.

At this point yon may get them to the shoulders in either of the following styles :—

Pull them up sharply towards the shoulders, with elbows pointing well out, splitting your feet back and forward, and sinking the trunk so as to get the shoulders down to the level with the bells, when by leaning sharply backwards you can exert such a pull as will greatly assist your arms in turning the bells to the shoulder.

This I think the best way, but some weight-lifters rise with the bells hanging at the sides, and then, swinging them first forward and then back, get a. good upward momentum towards the shoulders to assist their body dip. The legs must, of course, be split slightly before swinging and again just before the dip.

The shouldered position also varies with different lifters. The majority prefer to have their elbows close at their sides, hands slightly out from the shoulders, and bells turned so that the front spheres or discs approach each other.

Mr. Inch, however, considers the best position to be one in which the upper arm is nearly parallel with the shoulder and in continuation thereof, with the forearm bent back so that the bells practically rest on the shoulders themselves. In this position he keeps his back straight and jerks from the shoulders, as in the bar-bell lift. He claims this as a discovery, and as one which is distinctly preferable to the older methods.

He is very probably right, but I have not so far tested his method thoroughly, finding that I can still do better in the position to which I am accustomed, as already described.

I have failed to see any advantage in this method, but Mr. Inch has certainly increased his own powers at the lift by the discovery of this, so there may be a good deal in it.

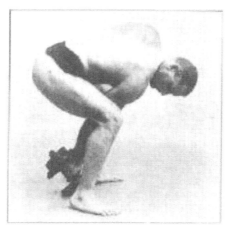

From either shoulder position the dumb-bells should be jerked aloft exactly as is the two-handed bar-bell.

If no restrictions be made about the bells actually resting on the shoulders and supported thereby, a far greater weight can be jerked by pulling them in and resting them on end on the shoulders as shown in illustration. The arms are then thrown straight, and by a slight body dip the correct position of a completed lift is obtained.

The Snatch

In getting into position for this lift, you will be posed as in the first stage of the single-handed clean lift to the shoulder, with the following differences :

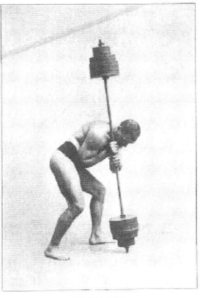

The Snatch.
Bringing the Bar-bell to the shoulder.

First, your feet may be slightly further apart (though it is true that most lifters make no alteration); secondly, your hands will be reversed (that is to say, the back of the hand snatching will be over the bar, instead of under it, and the little finger, instead of the forefinger, of your disengaged hand will be nearest your knee-cap); thirdly, you will bend over at the waist instead of at the hips; and fourthly, you will not bend so much at the knees.

33

Stand a moment with hand ready to snatch, before diving for the weight, gathering your energies. Then go down sharply, grip the exact centre of the bar (which you have, of course, previously marked), and pull up sharply with hand and shoulder, at the same time pressing hard on the left knee, so as to get the bell well aloft; when you dip rapidly at the knees and hips, into a sitting posture right under the weight, which may even be thrown a little back.

The arm should now be quite straight and an erect posture easily regained; but remember to use as many muscles as possible simultaneously in this lift—legs, both arms, and shoulder; pressing, pulling, and pushing as directed for each.

You can, if you like, instead of dipping underneath, sink beneath sideways, as in the bent press, to secure a straight arm, with the extra advantage of being able to assist with a slight final press, should the snatching arm fail to go quite straight at the first time of asking. This slight press is, of course, strictly speaking, illegal; but, at the same time, if it is but a very slight one and performed very quickly, it may easily escape notice.

The Two-handed Snatch

This lift is practically a clean bar-bell jerk all the way. The pull in is the same as in the two-handed bar-bell lift, but there is no stop. The moment it reaches the shoulder (or, rather, passes the head in this instance) the dip and jerk aloft follow instantaneously.

34

Both single and double-handed snatching will be found to be excellent practice for the single and double-handed clean pulls in, but it must be remembered that the arm, or arms, should not be bent in any way until the " turn " commences.

The Dumb-bell Swing
The only difference between this lift and the snatch is that the swinging hand is turned thumb to the front. The muscles employed therein are practically the same, and yet it does not follow that a record " snatcher " will always be a record " swinger."

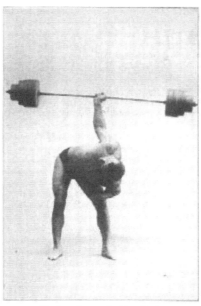

The Best Press on One Hand Press.
Showing how the elbow leaves the side and travels round to the back.
This is the most critical point of the lift.

In swinging the dumb-bell, the weight must be placed between the feet. The body then bends over from the waist, and a grip is taken of the bell close to the front sphere or disc. The bell may be rested on its end prior to swinging, and the disengaged hand should be pressed on the corresponding knee. Then with the head bent well down, swing the arm straight up, forcing the shoulders back, pushing with the thigh muscles and pressing with the disengaged hand.

Just as the force of your initial swing aloft is failing, dip beneath the bell and twist your wrist so as to get the arm straight, and rise immediately erect. Make the lift look as though it was a clean swing up as much as possible.

NOTE TO CHAPTER.—In all the lifts described in this chapter, and, indeed, throughout the book, always keep your eyes fixed on your weight so as to concentrate your mind on them, and endeavour always to anticipate your dipping movements. The second impetus to your lift, which you will derive from your said dips, must always be on hand and ready to come into action before the first impetus is fully expended.

NOTE re PULLING IN.—Many weight-lifters make the mistake of going about this in far too great a hurry, particularly when the weight is pulled in with both hands. Bring up your bell with a slowish steady pull. Make no attempt to rush it until just before the turn, then move like lightning, turn elbows as sharply as possible, and dip a little to help the bar to your chin.

CHAPTER III
The Bent Press

THIS lift, which more than any other is associated with my name, cannot be described as being either an English or a Continental lift. The two-handed lift to the shoulder is certainly akin to the Continental method of getting the weight into that position " anyhow," but the lift itself is not overmuch practised there.

On the other hand, the body press with one hand only, part of it is purely an English style of lifting, and one scarcely practised on the Continent at all, certainly not in the competitions.

Nevertheless, despite this, it is to my mind (and this quite apart from the successes I have achieved at it) one of the best feats, if not the very best, which has ever been devised. Strength, stamina, and science all enter into it in equal proportions, and the man who would make a success of the lift, a striking success that is, must necessarily be a first- class all-round lifter.

Those of you who have studied the lists of records published in the "Health and Strength Annual" cannot have failed to notice that the majority of world's record holders are distinguished for their feats at either one or a group of lifts, in which much the same muscles are called into play. That is to say, you will rarely find that a man who has eclipsed all rivals at a two-handed jerk or push has done much at single-handed lifting or snatching. In short, that these record holders are not as a rule all-round lifters.

For this reason, I would strongly advise one and all to make a special study of the " bent press," because it is an all-round lifter's lift; and I am firmly of the opinion that, in a match, an all-round lifter (not holding any records) would always defeat, more or less easily, a world-renowned record-holder, who had gained his fame simply and solely by virtue of his success at his one pet feat.

I have already described the final stages of the bent press in my remarks on the single-handed "clean all the way " lift, so have now only to deal with that portion of it in which the bell is lifted to the shoulder with both hands from an upended position.

To do this properly, the upright bell should be grasped with the right hand in the exact centre, the feet being well apart (if possible, exactly in the positions they will occupy throughout the lift). Fix the right elbow, resting firmly on the hip bone in front, and grasp the bell with the left hand, immediately below the right.

Bend well forward, leaning your head right over ; bend the legs well at the knees, and pull the weight over on to your shoulder.

In order to do this properly, you must lift strenuously with both hands, leaning well back and levering the bar over by the help of both your hip bones to secure and maintain your purchase, and of your shoulder, which you naturally slide as far as you can under the bar.

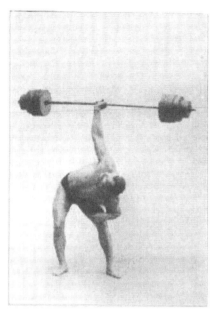

The hoist to the shoulder is rendered easier by the weight of the bell itself, the top sphere or discs being unsupported in any way, helping to pull the front sphere or discs upwards. A greater weight can be lifted by the bent press, if the bell be shouldered in one movement, since less energy is expended thereby; but if it will not come over at once, an additional heave becomes necessary. In order to avoid any necessity for two or three hoists (always exhausting) use as long a bar as is obtainable.

Once, however, it is fairly shouldered, the left hand can release its hold and be thrown out to adjust the balance, while the right, after steadying the bell, shifts round gradually, following the elbow as it slides round the hip bone to the back, into the proper position for the body press.

The method described above necessitates a fairly long bar for its perfectly correct performance, and other methods must be adopted with shorter ones.

The following, which may be also used with a long bar, if preferred (although I do not recommend such a procedure), is to place the feet as before (although they will very probably shift themselves subsequently in this instance), and having gripped the bar in the exact centre with the right hand, to again grip it with the left, but on this occasion close to the bottom sphere or disc.

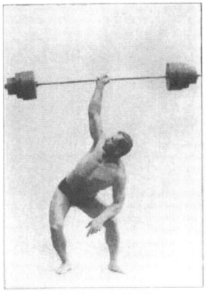

The Bent Press on One Hand Phase.
Tipped by sitting down before commencing to rise.

Bend the knees well and, pressing the bell against the body, with the right elbow away therefrom, lift the bell up and away from the body with the left hand. As soon as it swings clear, throw, jerk, or toss it in such fashion that you can slip your shoulder well under the bar.

On no account, now, leave go with your left until you feel that the weight is secure at your shoulder and your right elbow has gained its proper position, resting on your hip bone.

From the above it will be readily recognised that this lift is performed far more easily with a long bar than with a short one, since the second method of shouldering it (necessary with the shorter implement) imposes a pretty severe strain on the lifting muscles, owing to the lack of the fulcrum secured by the right elbow resting on the hip bone, as in the first method, and to the smaller assistance derived in overbalancing the weight.

One has only to study the further stages of the lift already described to realise that the lifting muscles need to be as fresh as possible, in order to cope satisfactorily with the press itself; and cannot afford to be strained in any way by the hoisting and tossing the bell to the shoulder, necessary with a short bar.

CHAPTER IV
The Continental Lifts

CONTINENTAL one-handed Weight-lifting records, apart from the snatch, the swing, and the weight held at arm's length, compare very unfavourably with English records. And naturally so, when it is considered how much more difficult the conditions are.

The bent press, for instance, is called "screwing" the weight, and rarely enters into the list of feats in an ordinary competition.

The Continental one-arm " press " is, in fact, almost a straight arm push from the shoulder, and might be described as such were there not an actual shoulder push as well, which I will describe later.

In the press, the bell is shouldered and then pressed (not jerked) to a straight arm, by arm strength only, no swing or jerk of the body being allowed, but the body may be- bent over slightly to one side. The legs also may be split slightly, to admit of the bending, but in these respects only does the lift differ from the one-handed push.

Continental One-Arm Push

This may be described as an arm press from the military position, i.e., from the ordinary position of a soldier at "attention." Heels together, toes pointing outwards, legs and back straight, and shoulders squared, the disengaged arm being allowed to be held slightly away from the body.

The weight itself is held level with the head, with the elbow close to the side, and must be pushed straight up by the use of the deltoid and triceps chiefly.

The world's record for this lift is, I notice, credited to Francois le Breton with 124 lbs.; but I have myself (although I have not devoted much attention to the lift) pushed 126 lbs. in this position, and have always understood that Michael Maier, of Vienna, once thus pushed 143 lbs.

Two-handed Bar-bell Continental Jerk

Here the Continental weight-lifters easily out-distance the Englishmen also, chiefly on account of the style in which they are allowed to lift. This time the advantage lies with them, since they are permitted to pull the bell in by a series of hoists.

The first of these pulls the bell up on to the abdomen in a clean lift with an over and an under grip, as shown in illustration. The bell is then lodged on the waist-belt (worn large for the purpose), while the left hand grip is changed to an over-hand one; then with a dip and a jerk it is hoisted on to the chest, and with yet another to the chin, preparatory to the final jerk which sends it aloft. Some even prolong this agony still further, making four, and sometimes five, jerks before they finally reach the chin.

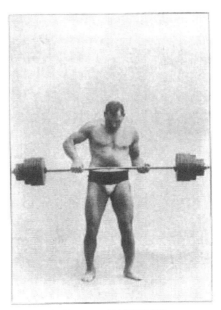

From that position it goes up as in the English jerk.

Wilhelm Tuerck, for instance, has jerked in this fashion 355 lbs., while Josef Steinbach has out-distanced even this feat. In fact, the latter's performances at this lift are so marvellous that his records deserve quoting in full.

On December 14th, 1905, he twice jerked 380¼ lbs.; on May 6th, 1905, he thrice jerked 350½ lbs.; on May 7th, 1905, he jerked 348¼ lbs. five times; and on October 8th, 1906, 330½ lbs. six times. All consecutive from the shoulders.

Two-handed Bar-bell Push

This also is a lift in which the weight is raised to the shoulders in a series of jerks, but from the shoulders must be pushed aloft by the arm and shoulder muscles chiefly, although with the legs split.

As being possibly of some interest to my readers, I have illustrated both Steinbach's and my own method of pushing a two-handed bar-bell. He, it will be seen, leans right back from the waist and pushes forward with his shoulders (as well as arms) in a diagonally upward direction. I, on the contrary, push with arm strength only from an erect position, with heels close together. Steinbach holds the record, but I cannot recommend his style. It suits him undoubtedly, but it appears to me to positively invite loss of balance, to say nothing of the risk of an unequal weight distribution.

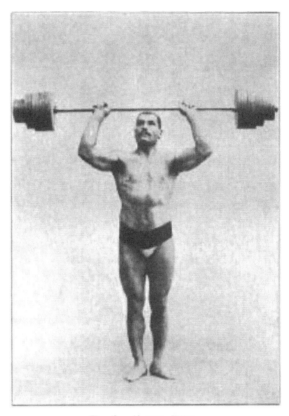

THE TWO HANDED PRESS,
(Continental Lift.) (Arthur Saxon's Style.)

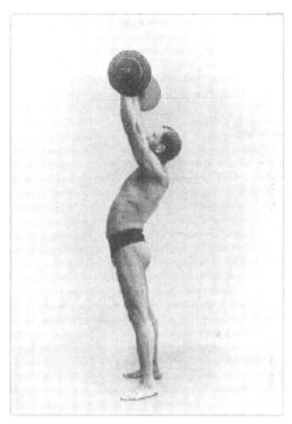

Two-Handed Bar-bell Press
(Josef Steinbach's Style)

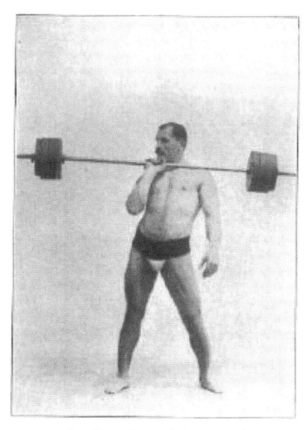

Bell Pulled In and Ready for Jerk.
(Continental Style)

Two Dumb-bells—Continental Style

These may be either pushed, by arm and shoulder strength only, as already described in the single and two-handed pushes, or they may be jerked as among English weight-lifters.

Steinbach, who has jerked a pair weighing 335 lbs. in all, holds the record, as he does in practically all two-handed lifts, save, of course, my own 448 lbs. get up anyhow.

In " pulling in" a pair of dumb-bells in the fashion adopted by him, the bells should be placed, first of all, between the feet; then, stooping down, they should be pulled up to rest on the thighs, after which, by leaning back and partly tugging them, partly heaving them from thence, you can get them on to your abdomen. A succession of jerks will then work them up your chest to your shoulders, when you must stand firm and collect yourself for the final jerk and dip which is to send them to arm's length above your head.

One-handed Jerk

This, also a lift which may be styled "Continental," is one at which my brother Hermann is particularly adept, his record being 210 lbs. Ai he lifts it, the bell is pulled in with over-hand grip in the " snatch " style, but only to the chin, where the arm being bent at the elbow, the bar rests, chiefly supported on the left shoulder, from which it is jerked aloft, the shoulder assisting considerably in throwing the weight up.

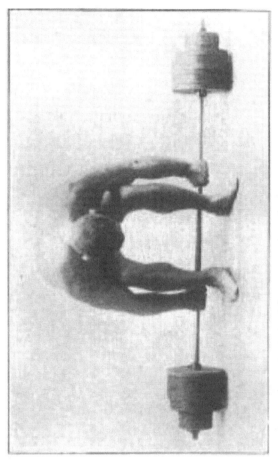

The Famous Barbell Dumbell and Kettle of the Book of the Bull Jointed. I. Pressing to put it.

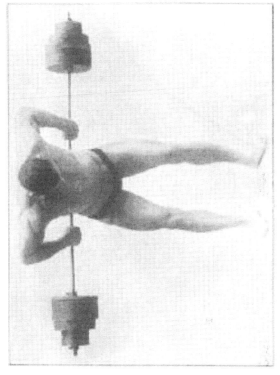

Two Minute Dumbbell Press and Roller Is Our Best Arm Thru Exercise

1) Pull up until upper end of bar, straightening the grip joints out and push to double.

51

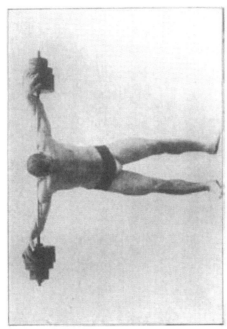

Two-handed Bar-bell rolled and pulled up the back, and then Jerked

This is a very effective lift, and not hardly so difficult as it looks or may appear at first.

Stand in front of, but close to, the bar, and grip it as shown in photograph, bending well forward from the waist. Pull the bar up smartly and rest it on the small of your back, straightening your legs as soon as you have done so. Now stooping forward, partly roll and partly pull it up your back till you arrest it at your shoulders, with the body nearly erect. Then quickly sliding your hands into position

No. 4, you are in the best position for a two-handed
jerk aloft.

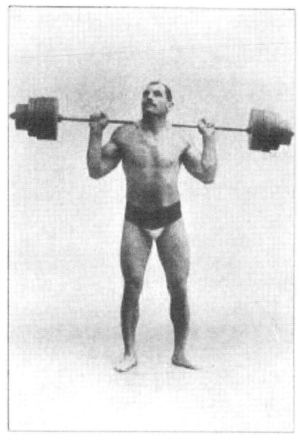

Two-handed Clean Press and Snatch Bar and Bell
Lifting.
No. 4. Best grip to jerk.

CHAPTER V
Ring, Ball, and Square Weight-lifting

IN Ring Weight-lifting the principal feat, of course, is to hold these out at arm's length. This can be done either in the English or in the Continental fashion, according to the rules governing the contest for which you are entered.

In the latter style the ring weight should be lifted and held palm downwards in front of the chest, with the arm (bent back at the elbow) horizontal with the shoulder. Then, turning the arm at the elbow, straighten it out horizontal with the shoulder. It is permissible to lean back a trifle, but must on no account overdo it.

In holding out weights right and left, a similar practice is observed (on the Continent) for each hand; but in England they can be raised to arm's length above the head, and then gradually lowered right and left until they are level with the shoulders —arms straight, palms being up on this occasion.

In holding at arm's length in front of one, the weight or weights should be raised from the ground until the knuckles are level with the eyes. The palm, or palms, should be turned down.

In lifting a ball or kettle-weight, the bell should be placed between the feet, handle parallel thereto. In pulling up, press off with disengaged hand from knee, as in single-handed lifts. As the ball passes the head, the foot corresponding to the lifting hand should stride out to the front, and the ball allowed to swing round to the back of the wrist.

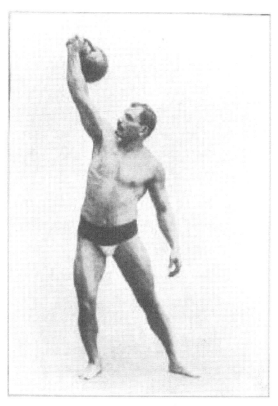

Be careful to let the ball swing round before the arm is fully extended, as in turning it with a straight arm, there is a risk of dislocating the wrist.

With square weights there is a very fair variety of lifts, which may be attempted. These may, for instance, be turned face to face and grasped round both handles with one hand, then pulled in and pressed. It is not possible to do anything very extraordinary in the matter of weight in this fashion, as the grip naturally presents considerable difficulty, but the lift is well worth practising for development purposes on that account alone.

Francois le Breton, the French weight-lifter, has put up some good feats in holding square weights at arm's length balanced on the palm of his hands. His records, which are well worth recording, are as follows : 77¼ lbs. at arm's length, right hand. Weights held out right and left, 143 3/8 lbs. in all, viz., 77¼ lbs. right and 66 1/8 lbs. left.

A Good Square or Ring Weight-lift

Here is a feat which, while never likely to be included in any competition, is well worth practising.

Get a square ring or kettle weight, such as you think you can manage. Tie a rope round the handle, and then twist it round your hand in such wise that when the arm is extended level with the shoulder, the palm turned to the front, the rope will be just taut.

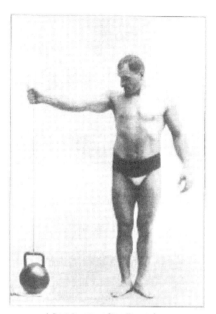

A Good Square or Ring Weight Lift.
Observe position of hand and arm. The arm to be quite rigid.

Now try and lift the weight from the ground in that position. I may mention that I have managed to raise 56 lbs. in this fashion, say half an inch, but the strain was tremendous. The rope must be taut, the arm horizontal with the shoulder, and the palm to the front before commencing. It sounds easy, doesn't it? Well, try the feat and see whether it is really so.

The accompanying photographs will show the positions, and the feat will be found an excellent exercise for developing strength.

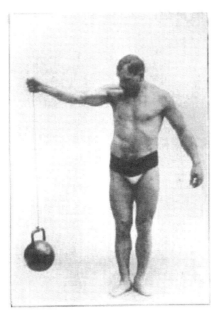

A Good Square or Bent Without Lift.
The weight should be lifted clean off the ground

CHAPTER VI
Weight-lifting Exercises and Exercises with Weights

AT first blush, these might seem to mean the same thing, but, as a matter of fact, there is a very considerable difference between the two.

A good many people imagine, when someone advises them to go in for a Weight-lifting course, that the only possible result will be to make weight-lifters of them.

Instead of which, as already mentioned in my first chapter, a series of Weight-lifting exercises will prove beneficial to any and every athlete, particularly from the point of view of cultivating and developing both health and stamina. They need not necessarily result in converting him simply and solely into a weight-lifter, although they will natur-ally tend to fit him for that occupation; they will, first of all, bring him into such a state of physical perfection as will enable him to compete successfully at almost any and every athletic pursuit, besides endowing him with as much health and stamina as he can possibly need for ordinary life.

Professor Inch, for example, has had athletes of every description through his hands, and adapts his lessons in accordance with their requirements.

Numberless professors of physical culture are continually propounding systems of exercise to the public, which they specially recommend on account of there being no necessity for any weights or other apparatus in their systems.

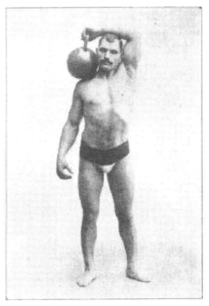

Front view Exercise No 6.
First position

I have nothing to say against these methods, as I have never tried them; but am perfectly satisfied, without troubling to investigate them, that only by exercising with weights can a thoroughly satisfactory all-round development be obtained. But, in order to secure this result, the exercising must be thorough, and it must be all-round. Each part of the body must be dealt with seriatim.

I proposed to set out in detail a list of exercises adapted to this end, but, on reflection, find that in order to do so I should need a book many times the size of this in order to accommodate the necessary illustrations; while in any case I should be giving little else than a duplication of the " Inch Advanced

Course." This last is the only thoroughly exhaustive system of Weight-lifting exercises with which I am acquainted, and is, moreover, one in which I had the pleasure of assisting to arrange.

There are, however, two arm exercises which I would like to recommend. It may, perhaps, be urged that these are really rather feats than exercises, although I personally practice them as exercises only.

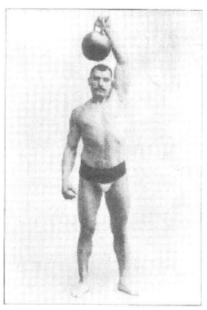

The first of these, which is a splendid arm exercise, particularly for the forearm muscles, is shown in an accompanying illustration. Stand as shown, with kettle-weight, say, 10 lbs., resting on the right shoulder, grasped with the left hand, the left arm being bent with forearm resting on the top of the head. Now straighten arm, raising the ball over your head and replace. Repeat ten to twenty times, with either arm, increasing number of repetitions gradually to, say, thirty times, then increase weight and commence afresh. The exercise may be varied by bringing the ball right over the head and resting it on the opposite shoulder, passing it all round the head, etc.

Another excellent arm exercise, which will be found to benefit the whole body, is also illustrated here. Care must, however, be taken in performing this, and as light a weight as possible used at first, which should be increased only gradually, unless the reader wishes to damage his face severely. Stand with feet apart, with kettle- weight, say 10 lbs., to commence with, on ground. Stoop down, and securing this with both hands, rise erect, bending the elbows and bringing the ball in line with mouth, taking care to keep the fingers close to the ball and arresting any possible backward swing of the ball with the thumbs, which should be placed as shown. Now thrust the ball to full arm stretch above the head, as shown in photograph, position 3. Return to No. 2 and then to No. 1. Repeat ten to twenty times, and increase as before.

Relaxing the Muscles

Always after exercising allow all the muscles to relax entirely and go absolutely limp. I do not anticipate that any of you will run clean through the whole series regularly every day, and, indeed, such a proceeding would be excessive. But the best plan to adopt is to decide which part of your body most needs development, and to adjust your exercises accordingly.

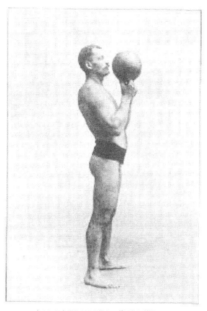

On no account, however, allow your backward groups to outstrip the promising ones by neglecting these latter entirely. Put in a spell at the exercises you don't think that you need every now and then, so as to ensure your regular all-round progress.

Always relax the groups exercised thoroughly, have a bath and rub down, and, if possible, get yourself well massaged all over before dressing again. Failing this, rub, stroke, pinch, slap, and pummel the muscles exercised so as to tone them up.

Finally, wear as little clothing as possible when exercising, and when in any doubt always consult some reliable and competent authority.

Exercises for Weight-lifting

If a man seriously proposes to go in for lifting heavy weights, he should make a point of practising certain lifts every day. This daily practice is absolutely essential to the achievement of any real success.

I have already stated that the surest method is to essay all-round lifting, and I would, therefore, recommend every aspiring weight-lifter to try and improve himself at every different feat.

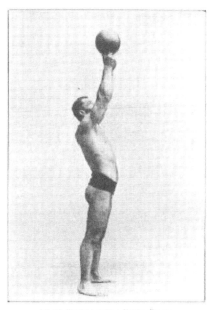

A Good Exercise with a Kettle Weight.
Hoist the bell to arm's length above the head.

Supposing him to possess a speciality however, with a fair chance of making a world's record thereat, ambition will, I have no doubt, overcome his good intentions in this respect, and will, consequently, impel him to devote more attention to his pet feat than it should properly receive.

Now, it is no manner of use preaching to deaf ears, so 1 will refrain from saying what I think of these would-be world's record makers, and will confine myself by imploring them to remember that such lifts as the snatch and the swing, for instance, will be excellent practice for both the jerk and the " clean pull in," and vice versa.

Just think carefully over the various lifts, and you will see that every lift develops particularly certain muscular groups upon which a very considerable strain is put in other lifts, which do not, however, test these same groups so severely.

It stands to reason, therefore, that the regular practice of all-round lifting must of necessity be excellent practice, not only for all-round lifting, but also for special and particularised lifting.

When you have let this sink into your minds, you can fairly easily ascertain your top weight in any particular lift, and can then devote your more special attention to increasing this limit. Carry on a similar process all-round, and the result cannot fail to be obvious to you.

One very useful trick which the weight-lifter should adopt is a wisely moderated contempt of his weights.

Don't despise them, for they are very formidable adversaries, and anything resembling overwhelming contempt will lead to failure.

But, nevertheless, it isn't a bad plan to write your weights down mentally. That is to say, supposing you are trying a 160 lbs. clean lift. Well, say to yourself, "Come, this is only 140 lbs., and I can lift it easily." Ten to one it will come up with an ease which will surprise you. That is, supposing you have " kidded " yourself properly and successfully.

Never on any account allow yourself to imagine that you are lifting heavier weights than you really are. If you must brag about your lifts, for heaven's sake, understate them.

It is the only safe plan, for the temptation to overstate, if submitted to, will become so strong as to master you yourself at last, and you will begin to fancy yourself such a hero as to be afraid of lifting at all for fear of proving yourself a liar.

CHAPTER VII
Exhibition and Trick Weight-lifting Feats

As previously hinted, the general public knows very little about Weight-lifting; that is to say, of either the science or art of it. They are far more impressed by the trickery which certain performers have seen fit to introduce.

Not that these performers are to be blamed for having adopted the course they have. They may or may not have possessed the necessary natural strength which would enable them to train on into becoming some of the strongest men in the world; certain is it that the effort, concentration and laborious practice necessary for the attainment of such a result would be to a large extent wasted effort, from a financial point of view.

The ordinary member of a music hall audience does not understand what real strength is. He is far more impressed by a performer who puts up a " swank" display, consisting of impossible feats (supposing these to have been really as advertised) than he is by the performance of genuine feats, transcending any previously achieved by any man.

For instance, I have seen the wildest enthusiasm lavished over the alleged performance of a feat (for which an elephant would not possess the necessary strength) by some performer who was unable to clean lift, say, 150 lbs.; and whose other physical powers were even less than would be illustrated by that comparatively insignificant feat.

Yet, for these reasons, it is always advisable for the weight-lifter to devote a certain amount of attention to the practice of exhibition and trick-lifting. Supposing him to have attained to any reputation, local or otherwise, he is certain to be asked to give a public display of his powers, at which, if he accedes, he will find that his best real feats, even though they be world's records, are accorded but a politely mild reception, save, of course, from fellow weight-lifters, who really know what he is doing.

But let him press a y stone man with one hand, and he will find that this feat is regarded as infinitely superior to a similar lift with a 250 lb. bar-bell. Let him lift the same man with his teeth, though it be only clear of the floor, and he will be regarded as a Hercules, a reputation which the two- handed jerk of a 300 lb. bell will not earn for him.

Let him, above all, trick seven or eight men, by telling them to push against a rod, which he is to hold rigid against their utmost efforts; and then, just as they are exerting their full powers, give it a small tug, which will cause them to fall face forwards in a heap, and the house will rise at him.

I have mentioned these few feats, because I have seen how well they have " gone down." The first two are genuine enough, and are worth practising on account of the effect they produce. Nor are they as easy as they sound. Even a 7 stone man is a pretty awkward object to press, though you may be able to manage fairly easily a 180 lb. bell. He is more difficult to balance and to hold securely. Then, again, he really needs to practice the role of human weight almost as carefully as you do that of human weight-lifter.

In working up such a feat, it is as well to remember that, for purely exhibition business, a stone or so will not make much difference in the spectator's mind. The average man is the poorest possible judge of another's weight. So a long, thin 8 stone man will often look heavier than a short, thick-set 10 stone one.

You may lift him, with your hand under the small of his back, in the pit of his stomach, or by gripping his upper arm (he having clasped his hands under his thighs).

A properly trained human weight will make this feat a comparatively easy one by springing up a little just as you commence to lift, the said spring to have been so well rehearsed as to be unnoticeable to the casual onlooker.

For exhibition purposes, again, the human weight can be introduced in various ways. It is not a bad plan to lift even a hollow kettle-weight to, say, shoulder height, and then to have your assistant lifted and seated thereon, when you press the combined weight to arms' length. The real weight of the man is of far less importance than his appearance, i.e., the weight he looks to be.

There are, of course, other methods in which human weights can be used. I have myself lifted and supported both my brothers, seated at opposite ends of a bar; but this is a real feat, and not one I should care to repeat too often.

Still, by utilising two 7 stone men, who, with the bar, will make a total press of less than 220 lbs., a man will achieve far more kudos, from the un-initiated, than he would by pressing even 300 lbs. of solid iron. Very few people are able to estimate the real weight of a bell cither by observation or by testing, and. in addition thereto, even actual knowledge that the bell does really weigh 300 lbs. or more would convey but little to their minds.

Similarly, the lifting of three, or even of two, 56 lb. ring weights is far more impressive to the ordinary man than a much heavier bar-bell. Most men are familiar with ring half-cwts., and know how awkward even one is to manage.

My own feat of supporting twelve men, seated on a plank, resting on the soles of my feet while holding up a heavy bell on which two other heavy men are seated, with my arms, has always taken well.

The mere fact that they are men, and not iron, proves to the audience that the feat is something out of the common far more convincingly than were I to support or press much heavier masses of iron.

This last-mentioned feat, by the way, reminds me of an exercise, necessary to practice, therefore. An exercise, moreover, which might well have been included in the last chapter.

I would, however, like; to warn my readers that tiny may encounter some really painful mishaps during their early acquaintance with it, but once the knack has been mastered, it will be found fairly easy, and besides, of immense value as a leg, back and neck developer.

Lie down on your back, with your legs raised at right angles to your body. Practice first of all pushing your body and legs straight up into the air, supporting yourself solely on your shoulders and the back of your neck.

When you have become proficient at this, lie down as before, pull a bar-bell (or even two ring weights) over your head, balance the first on the soles of your feet, or hang the second on your toes. Then straighten and bend your legs from ten to twenty times. Continue to practice this exercise until you have so strengthened the muscles, both of these and of your back, that you can press yourself, weights and all, up again on to your shoulders and back of your neck as before.

Continue this practice, increasing your repetitions once or twice every week, until you can perform the feat, say, twenty times in succession, when you should commence again, having increased the weight supported on your feet by 5 lbs. or so.

When commencing this leg and back strengthening exercise, it is advisable to use ring weights, as these are less liable to fall off, with painful consequences to yourself. Still, do not on that account avoid the exercise with a bar-bell as well, later on. Variations can be introduced with a bar-bell which are not possible with ring weights (such as men hanging on to the ends of the bar, etc.), while the weight raised can also be considerably increased.

As a last warning, I would recommend that when using a bar-bell, it would be as well to cultivate the knack of pitching the bell away from you, once control is felt to be going. A quick jerk of the feet will be all-sufficient for this, and you will avoid the extremely unpleasant consequences incident to the bell rolling off on to you yourself.

9581502R00043

Printed in Great Britain
by Amazon.co.uk, Ltd.,
Marston Gate.